Letter from the Publisher

Amanda Klenner

Viola odorata, or Violet: a beautiful name for a beautiful lady. This is one of the first herbs to peek up when the weather starts to warm, the snow melts, and the plants begin to regain some of their vibrant nature after the cold winter. The beautiful leaves are hidden in lawns and ride low in the planes and on forest floors, hardly seen unless a person is looking to find them. Once you locate violet, you might find that it is spread far and wide. It is a common "weed" that spreads plentifully in lawns, gardens, and fields.

The beautiful purple flowers are shy and hard to see, hence the expression, "shrinking violet," used to describe a shy person. Indeed, myths abound, lending to this common herb an air of intrigue. Violet is considered the flower of modesty and virginity, often associated with the Virgin Mary. In Victorian floriography ("the language of flowers"), violet was a symbol of retiring modesty, which has led to its status as the flower to give for a 50th wedding anniversary.

Not surprisingly, this popular flower also has historical use as a medicinal plant, but is often overlooked in modern pharmacopeias. Although not many studies have been done on the medicinal benefits of violet, thousands of years of use by traditional healers is not to be discounted. I personally use violet to add some moisture and demulcent action to highly astringent and drying preparations like red raspberry leaf, nettle leaf, and sage. Violet's flavor is "green," which usually indicates a high mineral content. It certainly adds support for the whole body.

Please enjoy this beautiful but overlooked herb, and let us know what you learn in our online forums or our Facebook page!

Table of Contents

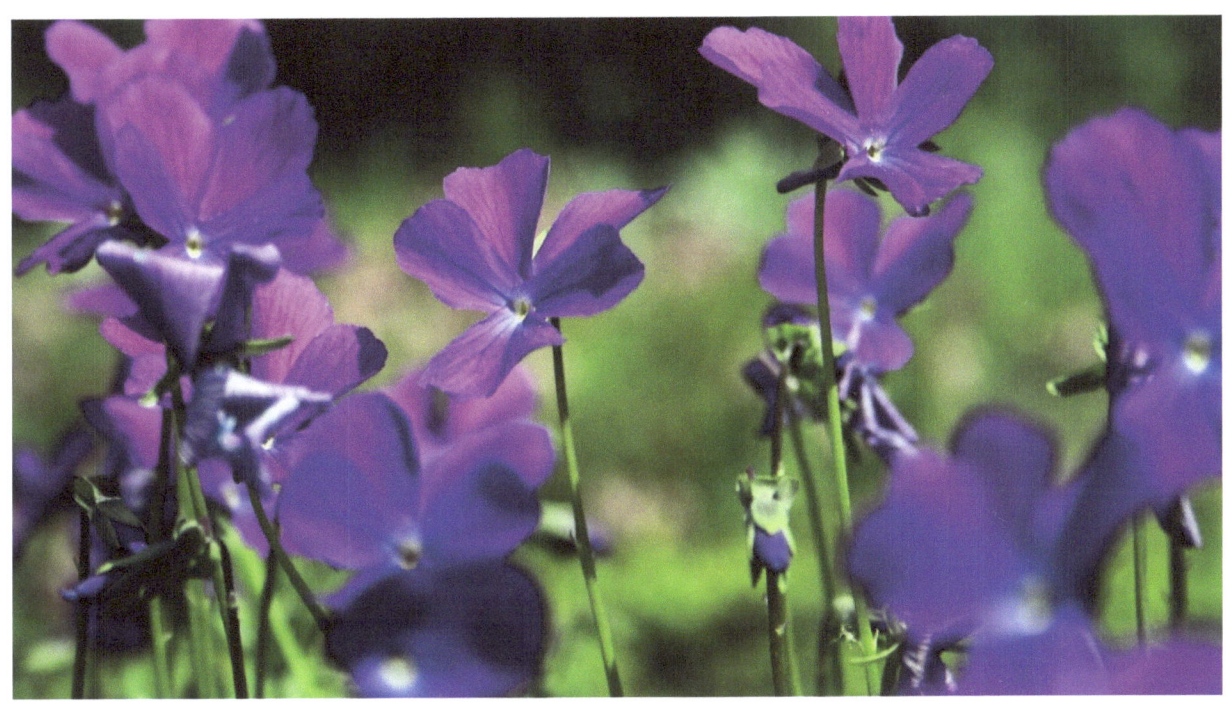

Violet Herbal Monograph

Angela Justis

Latin Name: *Viola odorata, Viola tricolor, and Viola spp*.

Family: Violacaea

Common Name: violet, sweet violet, shy violet, viola, wild pansy, heartsease, pansy, Johnny-jump-up

Parts Used: primarily leaves and flowers

Flower and Leaf Actions: refrigerant, demulcent, nutritive, expectorant, lymphagogue, alterative, discutient, anodyne, vulnerary, antiseptic, emollient, laxative, anti-inflammatory, anti-rheumatic, anti-neoplastic, diuretic

Root Actions: emetic, cathartic, expectorant, antipyretic

Constituents: mucilage, saponins, salicylates, vitamin A, vitamin C, antioxidants, phytosterols, quercetin, essential oils

Description: *Viola odorata* and other *Viola* species grow in moist, shady areas but will spread into lawns and gardens as well. Often found in grouped masses, the plants grow close to the ground. While budding, the little flowers hide beneath heart-shaped green leaves. The asymmetrical flowers have five petals—two on top, two on the side, and one at the base of the flower, with a tiny yellow center. Blossom color ranges from deep purple to yellow to white, or even combinations of the three. Once in full bloom, the flowers appear above the leaves. The flowers have a distinctive and heavenly scent, especially those of the common violet species, *Viola odorata*. The leaves are a bit downy (fuzzy-fluffy). They roll in at the edges when they're young, and as they age, they become flatter.

Violet's Many Uses

She is calling, and her delightful scent wafts through the air, announcing spring's arrival. Violet's tiny, vivid, purple flowers are all full of beautiful fragrance and good medicine. This lovely little plant only flowers for a short while each spring, truly an ephemeral gift from the Earth.

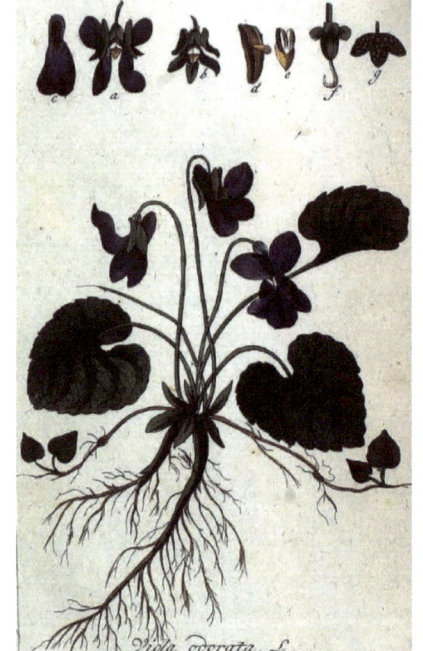

The beloved violet has been revered throughout the ages. Its sweet beauty symbolizes modesty, fertility, and love, while the plant itself finds use as a medicine for the heart, respiratory system, and more. This tiny, unassuming plant is gentle but powerful medicine.

Nourishing Violet

Violet is full of delicious nutrients! Traditionally used as a nutritive food, it's a superbly nourishing vitamin-rich plant that eases and soothes with its gentle mucilage. Specifically, violet leaves and flowers are high in vitamins C and A. According to Susun Weed, "A cup of violet infusion supplies 6,000 IU of carotenes,"[1] while "100 grams of fresh spring leaves contain 264mg of ascorbic acid and 20,000 IU of vitamin A."[2]

Use violet leaves to make delicious salads and soups. The flowers are beautiful as a special garnish on salads, cakes, and cookies. They can also be preserved through crystallization and used as a cheerful decoration during the long winter. (See Erin's article on page 35 for all manner of culinary inspiration!)

A Child's Friend

Violet is an excellent children's herb. The enchanting little flowers and softly fuzzed, heart-shaped leaves are so fun to play with! The flowers and leaves make a yummy little snack when kids are playing outside on a happy spring day; and they can use the flowers to make a gift for the fairies, or to decorate salads and cookies.

Another favorite project for kids is making violet honey. The delightful floral flavor of violets combined with sweet, golden honey is delicious to enjoy by the spoonful, drizzle on biscuits and toast, or to sweeten a cup of tea. (See Erin's recipe for violet honey on page 40.)

All this fun, and violet may also lend a hand when children aren't feeling well, too. A cough syrup made from the flowers and/or leaves (see page 31) has long been used to soothe away childhood coughs and scratchy throats, while the leaves and flowers together can help cool inflammation and fever, plus ease associated aches and pains.[3] Violet flower syrup is also commonly used to settle children's stomachaches, acting as a gentle laxative in cases of constipation.[4] Heartsease (*Viola tricolor*) is known as a home remedy for cradle cap in babies.[5]

Cooling Soother

A compassionate friend, violet is thought to support the heart, helping people through times of grief and heartache, providing comfort and strength.[6] A sweet little poem from Earnest Leaverton's 1919 book, *In the Garden of the Heart*, reminds us that violet's purpose it to "gladden the heart of a sprite like you."[7]

Violet leaf consumed as an infusion or applied topically as a compress or poultice can ease the pain of headaches and tension by gently dissipating heat while supporting the body and the nerves.[8,9] Furthermore, violet has been used to clear heat from the head related to nervousness, fever, and infections. This pretty, unassuming little plant supports cooling sleep, especially easing a restless mind and a sad heart.

Violet has also been useful in easing the pain and inflammation of arthritis and rheumatism, nourishing the body while reducing the heat of inflammation and moistening and lubricating the tissues, providing relief from dryness.[6] Masterfully stated by herbalist Kiva Rose, "Something I adore about Violets is their gentle, but thorough nature. For cooling, calming, lymph moving, pain relieving kind of action this flower is a master."[10] These wonderful qualities find use in many conditions.

Violet is perfect for gently but powerfully clearing congested lymphatic states. An infusion (tisane) taken internally has been known to help at the beginning of illness when the nodes are tender and warm. Used externally, as an infused oil or poultice, it may also assist in clearing chronically stuck lymph.[11]

Violet is a cooling, moistening expectorant that soothes respiratory ailments such as bronchitis, whooping cough, and flu—in particular those associated with irritable coughing and thick, yellow catarrh.[6] For adults and children alike, the slippery, soothing quality of violet has long been known to help relieve sore throats. Jim McDonald cleverly recommends "keeping a wad" of fresh leaf in your cheek to take advantage of the mucilage for a sore throat.[11] This mucilage, along with violet's antiseptic action, can also help in cases of urinary discomfort such as cystitis and infections.[12]

Sisterly Love for Women

For women, violet may offer healing sisterly love, decreasing swelling and soreness in breast tissue, for instance in mastitis, fibrocystic breasts, PMS, lumps, and cancer. For nursing mothers suffering with cracked nipples, a soothing violet poultice can bring welcome relief and healing. Violet oil is a beautiful choice for breast care.2 (See Jessica's recipe for breast lotion on page 21, or Jan's breast balm recipe on page 27.)

Herbal Cancer Ally

Long used to dissolve and heal lumps in the body, violet leaf infusions, oil, and poultices have a reputed history of use for helping those dealing with cancer of the breasts, lungs, lymphatic glands, urinary tract, and GI tract.[2,3,14] There is perhaps no greater proponent of violet's usefulness in fighting cancer than renowned Herbalist Susun Weed, who considers a violet poultice to be "especially invaluable when dealing with *in situ* carcinomas."[15] Weed further states, "internal and external use of violet can shrink a breast lump in a month."[16] She also believes that violet has the ability to slow cancer growth and relieve "the pain in cancerous growths, especially in the throat."[14]

Aside from helping those with cancer, violet can be an essential addition to any longevity lifestyle. In her book *Breast Cancer? Breast Health!*, Susan Weed encourages us to use violet as part of an anti-cancer lifestyle. She explains that high amounts of phytochemicals present in plants like violet help keep us healthy and nourish the immune system, supporting the body in keeping cancer at bay.

External Uses

As an external remedy, violet leaf can be invaluable for healing hot, inflamed skin issues. A poultice, oil, or wash may help to heal fresh abrasions as well as more persistent purulent wounds. Violet, probably due to its antiseptic and vulnerary actions, is also quite commonly used to clear pimples and abscesses. And, as I mentioned earlier, it has been used topically as an oil or poultice to dissolve lumps. It can be used both internally and externally for helping ease more chronic issues such as eczema and herpes, as well as other scaly skin conditions.[4,17] A gentle wash made with violet is thought to soothe sore eyes.

Getting to the Root

Violet's roots are strong medicine indeed and should be used by skilled herbalists as they can cause stomach distress as well as issues with breathing and blood pressure. Similarly to the leaves and flowers, the roots have been used to cool and clear issues with respiratory illness.

Using Violet Safely

We always have to consider that herbs are medicine, and as such, must be regarded with concern for safe dosage, how they may interact with other medicines, and how they can affect individuals with certain illnesses or sensitivities.

Safety Considerations

No dangerous interactions with violet are known, but always check with a doctor or clinical herbalist if you have any questions about its use with other medicines. In large doses, the roots can cause extreme stomach upset and issues with breathing and blood pressure regulation. The leaves may cause an allergic reaction such as itchiness, burning, and "minor eruptions"[18] People who are allergic to violet should avoid using it medicinally.

Preparation and Dosage

Here are the various ways you can prepare violet, along with some dosage guidelines.

Infusion: Prepare the leaves and flowers as an infusion left to steep for 4 to 8 hours, and drink freely.

Tincture: *Viola tricolor* 30 to 40 drops, 2 to 5 times per day for adults. Use Clark's Rule to adjust for children.[19]

Syrup: 1-5 tsp per day of violet syrup (see page 31). Take just before bed for insomnia.[4]

Topical Preparations: Prepare as a wash, poultice, or oil and apply as needed, increasing frequency with acuteness of the situation.

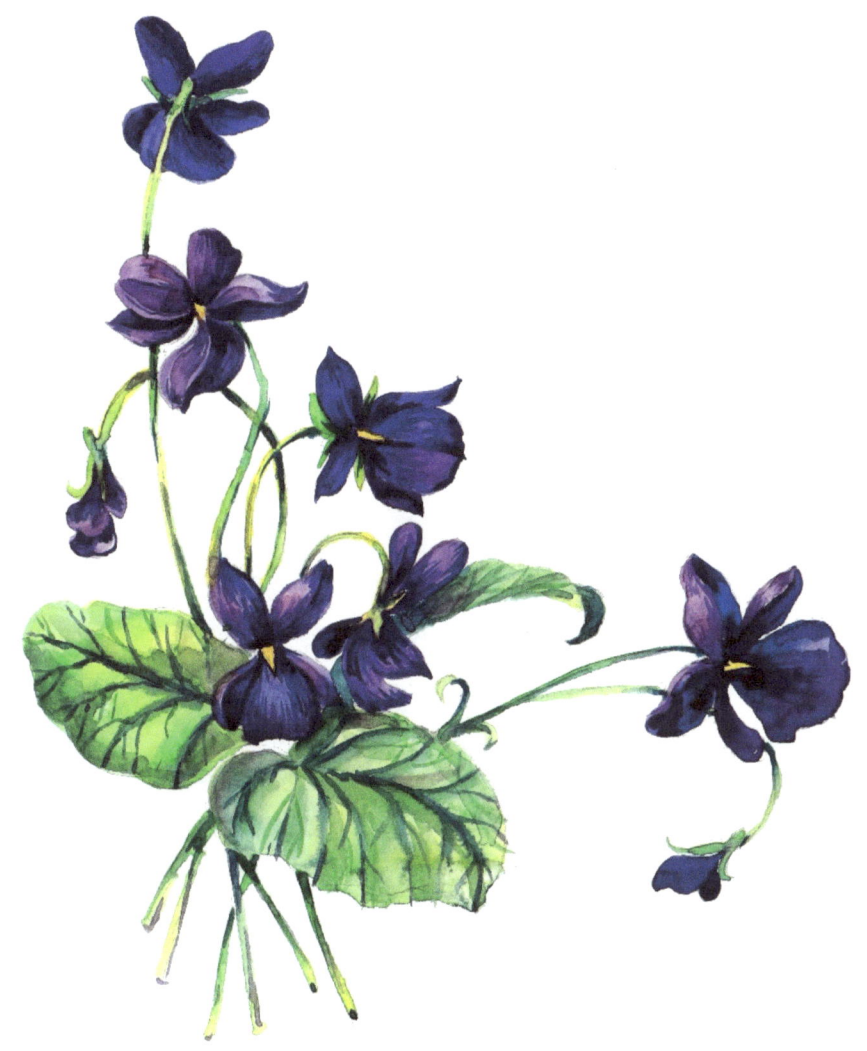

The History of Violet

Stephany Hoffelt

Transformation

Few flowers have a more interesting history than the violet. The oldest myth concerning violets is of Phrygian origin. In this story, the great mother goddess Cybele loved a hunter who was gored to death by a wild boar. His blood transformed to violets as it fell to the ground.

The theme of transformation surrounding violets persisted for centuries. A Roman myth tells that Jupiter first caused violets to appear for Io to graze on, after she had transformed to a white heifer. The ancient Romans associated violets with the love goddess Venus due to a myth that she jealously beat some young maidens blue and they transformed to violets. A Romanian folktale tells the story of a young girl who is abandoned in a deep forest to freeze to death and survives by becoming a violet. In the 16th century, French poet Nicolas Rapin wrote that the first violet was a beautiful young nymph whom the goddess Diana transformed into a flower to save her from Apollo's unwanted advances.

Ceremony

Violets have also been a ceremonial plant since ancient times. The Romans believed that the nymph Chloris accompanied the sun, scattering roses, violets, and lilies in its wake; and many of their rituals, particularly Rosalia, included strewing violets and roses. The Greeks, especially he Athenians, frequently employed the little purple flowers to make garlands and chaplets for use in rituals. Violets were so popular in Athens that the Greek playwright Aristophanes dubbed Athens the "Violet-Crowned City." The mythology explains that this is because the founder of Athens, Ion, was given violets by water nymphs in order to entice him to settle near them.

There are many historical references to violets as a funerary flower as well. It is the violet's association with mourning which led to the color purple being associated with Lent, in Catholic rituals. The first stories speak of violets springing up on the graves of virgins and saints, leading to Shakespeare's Laertes saying of Ophelia, "Lay her in the earth, / And from her fair and unpolluted flesh / May violets spring." Tennyson also alludes to this theme when commemorating his friend Arthur Henry Hallam: "And from his ashes may be made, / The violet of his native land." In Wales, violets were only planted on the graves of infants who had died.

Art and Literature

Violets pop up frequently in European history. During the Renaissance, the Virgin Mary was frequently painted holding violets, as in Leonardo da Vinci's *Madonna and Child with Flowers*. In France, a golden violet was given to the author of the best poem at the Toulouse festival. When Napoleon went in to exile, his followers dubbed him "La Pere la Violette" and wore or hung small sprays of violets to show their support of him. When his wife Josephine died, he covered her coffin in violets. In Germany, the folk dance *Alter Reigen um das erste Veilchen* celebrates the first violets of spring.

The violet has been perhaps most enthusiastically embraced in the UK. From medieval times on, the violet figured heavily in their literature and customs. In *A Handful of Pleasant Delites*, published in 1584, Clement Robinson wrote:

> Violet is for faithfulnesse,
> Which in me shall abide;
> Hoping likewise that from your heart
> You will not let it slide.

Two centuries later, Scottish bard Robert Burns wrote, "The violet's for modesty, which weel she fa's to wear, / And a' to be a Posie to my ain dear May."

Custom

The Victorians were mad about violets. They considered the blue violet a symbol of both modesty and faithfulness, due to the flower's literary history. The white violet was associated with virtue and happiness. Street vendors sold little bouquets, which would often then be tucked into small bouquets, known as Tussie Mussies, to convey these sentiments to someone they admired.

Cuisine

The violet has long and regal culinary history in the UK. Medieval monks made a cordial of *Viola tricolor*, which they served to honored guests. King Edward was fond of violet sugar, which is made simply by putting alternating layers of violet petals and sugar in a jar and setting the jar aside for a few weeks.

Simple Sugared Violets

During Queen Elizabeth's reign, she liked to have crystallized violets to flavor her deserts and as edible garnishes. While there is a more difficult crystallization process that involves boiling the petals in sugar, you can easily substitute simple sugared violets. Try them as a garnish on a rich vanilla custard!

Ingredients

- 2 C violet petals
- Egg white of 1 large egg, at room temperature
- 1 tsp water
- 1 C superfine sugar

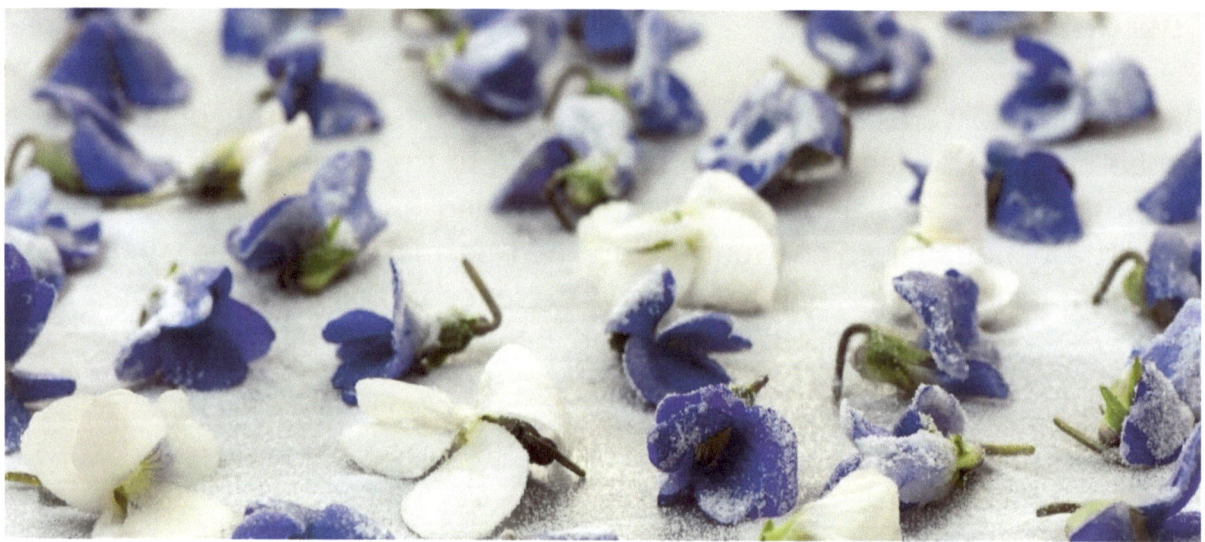

Directions

1. Rinse and dry the flowers.
2. Preheat the oven to 180 degrees. Alternately, you can use a dehydrator set to its highest setting.
3. Whisk the egg whites until frothy, slowly adding in the water.
4. Use a small paintbrush to gently paint this mixture onto both sides of the flowers' surface.
5. Lightly coat each petal with sugar, being sure to shake off any excess. You still want to be able to see the color(s) of the flower.
6. Place the sugar-painted flowers on a baking sheet covered with parchment paper or a dehydrator tray.
7. When you're done with all the petals, turn the oven off and leave the baking sheet in the oven to sit overnight. If using a dehydrator, you will want to keep an eye on the petals. You want them to retain their color, so take care not over process them.

Violet Jelly Recipe

Violet petals were considered a delicacy in the Victorian era. They were used to make cakes, syrups and jelly. A favorite dessert was violet wafers served with lemon balm sauce. Violet jelly was often served at teatime with sweet cream scones.

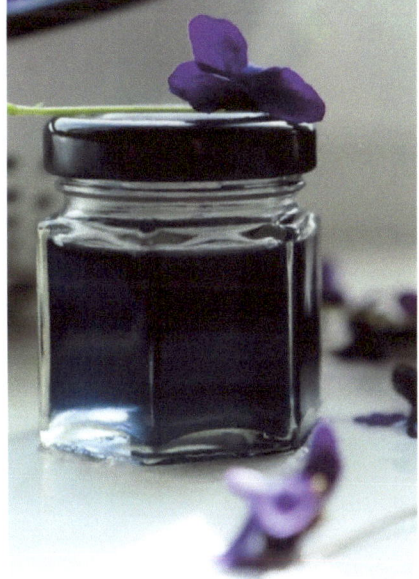

Ingredients

- $2\frac{1}{2}$ C fresh violet petals
- 2 C boiling water
- $\frac{1}{4}$ C lemon juice
- 4 C sugar
- 3 ounces liquid pectin

Directions

1. Prepare your jars, lids, and rings by washing them and sterilizing them in boiling water.
2. Wash the petals and place them in a glass container with a tight-fitting lid.
3. Pour the boiling water over the flowers and cover the container. Let this sit overnight.
4. Strain the liquid through a fine sieve. It should be a dark blue-green color.
5. Add the lemon juice. The liquid will turn to a more purple color.
6. Place this liquid and the sugar in a stainless steel saucepan.
7. Bring the liquid to a rolling boil; stirring frequently to make sure all your sugar is dissolved.
8. Add the liquid pectin and boil for 3 minutes. If the mixture foams, skim the foam from the top.
9. Ladle the mixture into prepared jars. Place the lids and rings on the jars.
10. Process in a hot-water bath for 12 minutes.
11. Remove the jars from the hot-water bath and allow them to cool. You should hear the lids pop, to indicate that they have sealed.

Only white sugar is going to give you a pretty purple jelly. If you use evaporated cane juice or sucanat, the recipe will work, but the jelly will not be as colorful.

This jelly is so delicious on scones or biscuits and contains a good deal of rutin, which is a flavonoid known for strengthening blood vessels.

I hope this little glimpse into the history of violets will inspire you to research more about its amazing history, or at least to make something yummy!

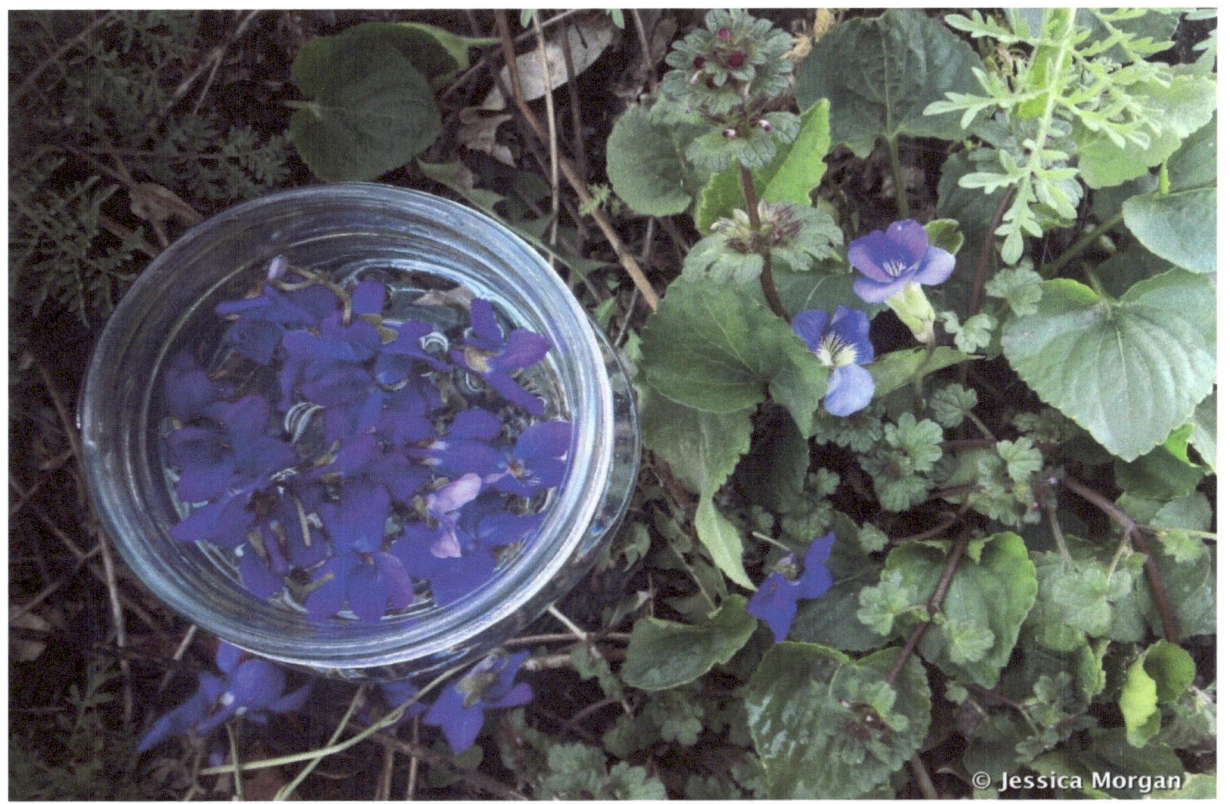
© Jessica Morgan

Cleansing Spring Violet Cream

Jessica Morgan

I'm fairly certain that every herbalist, gardener, and plant lover alike rejoices when the wild violets start springing up in the spring. Their adorable heart-shaped leaves and dainty little carpet of purpley-blue is definitely a sight for sore eyes!

Over here in Colorado, they're also one of the first flowers to bloom in spring and I simply can't get enough of their farewell-to-winter cheer. As pretty as they are, violets aren't just a purple-flowered weed; yes, they're cute with their charming pop of color, but they're also edible and add a fresh, vibrant sweetness to foods. Plus, they're medicinal—what could be better? Moreover, violets aren't really shy, even though they may act it. You can find them just about everywhere, as long as you look. So go on, get down in the grass, under the trees, and behind other plants….start looking and picking…and nibbling!

"I think it pisses God off if you walk by the color purple in a field somewhere and don't notice it." ~ Alice Walker, The Color Purple

Violet, with her dark, heart-shaped green leaves, fancies the shade and purposely grows under the protective straight of the trees, around other flowers, and within the grasses, which gives her the confidence to bloom. It is said that violet flower essence is uplifting and imparts feelings of joyfulness that can be experienced as lightness, as if sparkling bubbles of light gently lift us off the ground, yet at the same time, grounding and aligning the body and energy center, giving us the confidence to bloom too.

All *Viola spp.* are edible and have similar medicinal value. The leaves, buds, and flowers can be eaten and are loaded with vitamins and minerals, especially A and C. You can eat them raw or cooked, but the flowers are most often added to salads or desserts as a garnish.

Medicinally, violet has an affinity to the lymphatic system, is classified as an alterative, or blood purifier, and is thought to promote the body's own cleansing action. It's also an effective anti-inflammatory, emollient, demulcent, and nutritive herb. It's known for treatment of swollen glands and helping the body to eliminate bacteria and other toxins, which is why violets are traditionally used in body and breast care. It's also used for chapped and dry spots. I love making a variety of face and body creams with both the leaves and the flowers.

Violet and Stinging Nettle Breast Cream

Here's one of my favorite lusciously clean-smelling creams, perfect for thirsty skin and for breast care. It's light, creamy, dreamy, and filled with the essence of spring violets. Make a batch and gift some to the women in your life! It's a great aid for mastitis, fibrocystic breasts, cysts, and to help shrink tumors and cancers. Whether you use a simple infused oil or the cream below, regular breast massages with violet can help keep breast tissue healthy and lump-free!

Ingredients

- 3 ounces violet-leaf- and nettle-infused sunflower oil (see instructions below)
- $^1/_2$ ounce castor oil
- $1^1/_2$ ounces shea butter
- $^1/_2$ ounce grated beeswax
- 2 vitamin E capsules
- About 1 C fresh violet flowers
- 1 C just-boiled water
- 5–8 drops ylang-ylang, jasmine, neroli or essential oil of choice

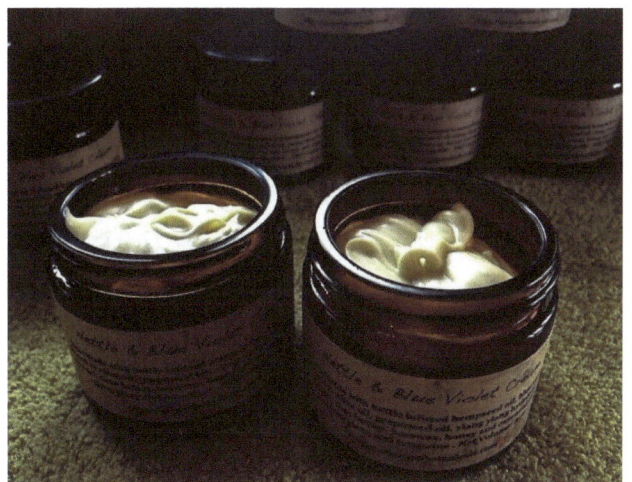

Infused Oil Directions

1. Lightly place dried or freshly wilted and finely chopped violet and nettle leaves into a completely dry jar. (It's important to cut the herb first to expose more of the plant to the oil, making for a better infusion.)
2. Fill the jar almost to the brim with oil, as an air gap will promote oxidation and spoilage.
3. Stir the contents with a chopstick until all the bubbles have dispersed, and cap it with a lid or a piece of cheesecloth and rubber band. (The cheesecloth works well for fresh plant material because it allows moisture to escape.)
4. Label!
5. You can leave it to infuse on a bright sunny windowsill or in a nice warm spot, like beside the boiler.
6. Stir every few days for the first 2 weeks, and then leave it to infuse uninterrupted for another 2 to 4 weeks.
7. Strain the oil through a sieve covered in cheesecloth or a jelly/paint bag.
8. Bottle the resulting oil, label and date!

Cream Directions

1. Now that you have your oil, you can begin making the cream. Place the 1 C of fresh violet flowers into a small heat-proof glass jar.
2. Pour the heated water over them, cover the jar, and let it steep while you carry out steps 3–8. This will make a violet tea.
3. Measure out your violet-leaf- and nettle-infused sunflower oil into a heat-proof measuring cup.
4. Add the castor oil, shea butter, and beeswax to the oil.
5. Set the cup into a shallow pan filled with several inches of water.
6. Heat on low until everything melts together. This will happen quickly.
7. Remove the measuring cup from the pan and let it cool to body temperature.
8. Add the vitamin E capsules. (I just poke a hole in the end of each capsule, squeeze it out, and then toss the gel cap.)
9. Strain the violet flower tea and measure out 5–6 ounces of it. (Don't forget to compost all the herbs!)
10. Get the oil and water to around the same temperature, either by heating one and/or letting one cool.
11. Using a hand mixer (or blender) on low, slowly drizzle the violet flower tea into your oil mixture while you blend the two liquids together.
12. As the mixture starts to thicken, increase the speed to high. Beat or blend it on high until it's is thick and creamy.
13. Stir in your desired essential oils.
14. The cream will continue thickening as it cools.
15. Spoon the cream into a clean, sterilized jar or tin, label it, and enjoy! Use generously and daily.

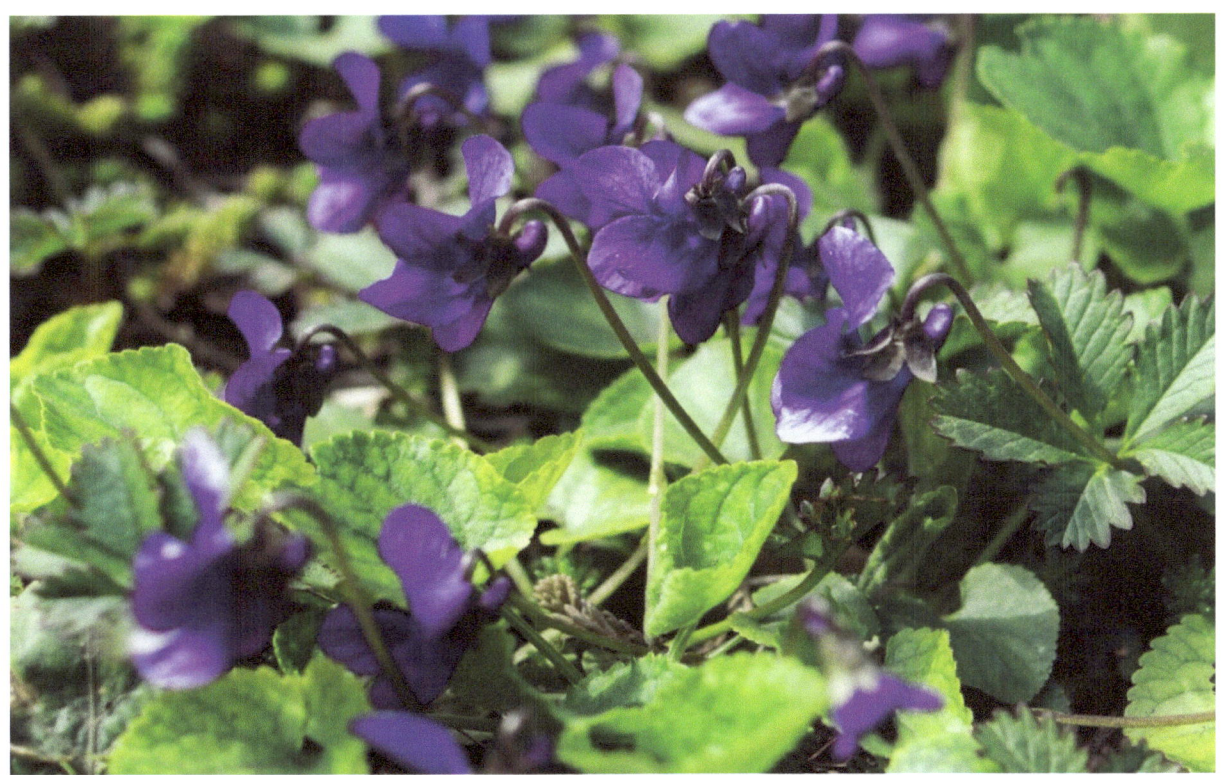

Violet Leaf for Breast Health

Jan Berry

Several years ago, I discovered a lump in my breast, made all the more worrisome since my mother and grandmother had both suffered from pre-menopausal breast cancer. After fretting over it for a while, I went to see my naturopath, who checked my blood and sent me for a thermographic scan. Everything came back fine, and I was diagnosed as simply having a mild case of fibrocystic breast disease.

While researching the condition, I came upon writings by the wise and wonderful herbalist, Susun Weed, which suggested using violet as an ally for breast health.

I read that violet is a lymphatic tonic that helps clear blockages and restore normal lymph flow. Fresh violet leaves have long been used as a poultice for reducing lumps and cysts in the breast, or infused into a massage oil for similar benefit.

Violet also contains anti-inflammatory properties, that can help ease the pain and discomfort that comes along with fibrocystic disease.

Since I had a yard full of violets and no extra money on hand for the other natural treatments my naturopath had in mind, I gave it a try.

I gathered handfuls of fresh violet leaves and dried them in single layers on clean dish towels for 2 or 3 days. I then turned the freshly dried leaves into an infused oil and applied it religiously each night. The oil proved to be a little messy to handle, but that problem was remedied by adding a small amount of beeswax to make it into a balm instead.

After a week or two of diligent use, I was happy and relieved to notice the discomfort fading away. These days, I only use it once or twice per week for maintenance and general breast health. I've also since added dandelion and calendula flowers to some batches, for their potential cancer-fighting and lymph-moving qualities.

Violet Leaf Oil

Making your own violet leaf oil is a simple process; and you can keep it as-is, or you can make it into a balm like I eventually did.

Ingredients
- About $1/2$ pint-jar of dried violet leaves
- $1/4$ pint dried calendula flowers and/or dandelion leaves (optional)
- 1 pint light oil, such a sunflower or olive

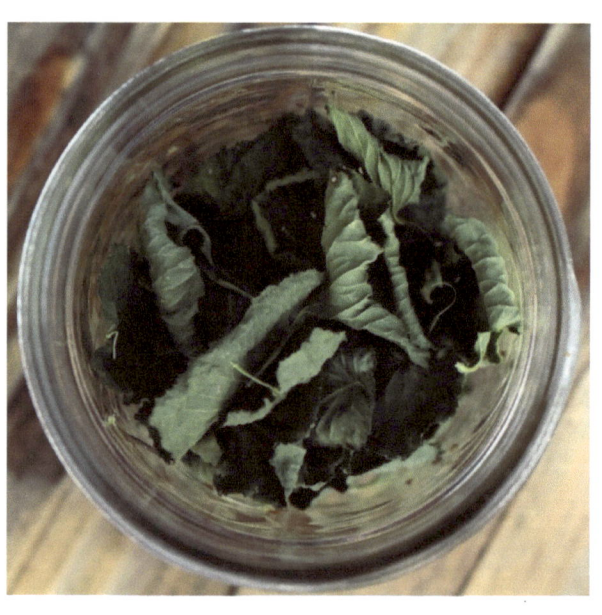

Directions
1. Put the herbs in a 1-pint glass jar.
2. Cover the dried herb(s) with the oil until it reaches the top of the jar, leaving an inch or so of space.

3. Stir a few times to get any trapped air bubbles out.
4. Cap the jar and set it aside for 4 to 6 weeks, shaking it occasionally to allow the healing properties of violet leaves to permeate the oil.

   Note: If you're in a hurry, you can speed up the infusing process by setting the uncapped jar down into a saucepan containing a few inches of water, forming a makeshift double boiler. Set the pan over a medium-low burner for around 2 or 3 hours, keeping a close eye on it so the water doesn't evaporate out.

5. Once the oil has infused to your satisfaction, strain and store it in a clean, dry jar. The oil will have a shelf life of about a year, if stored out of direct heat and sunlight.

Violet Leaf Breast Balm

Once your oil is infused, you can use it to make the balm, which is much easier and cleaner to apply than the oil! (All measurements are by weight.)

Ingredients

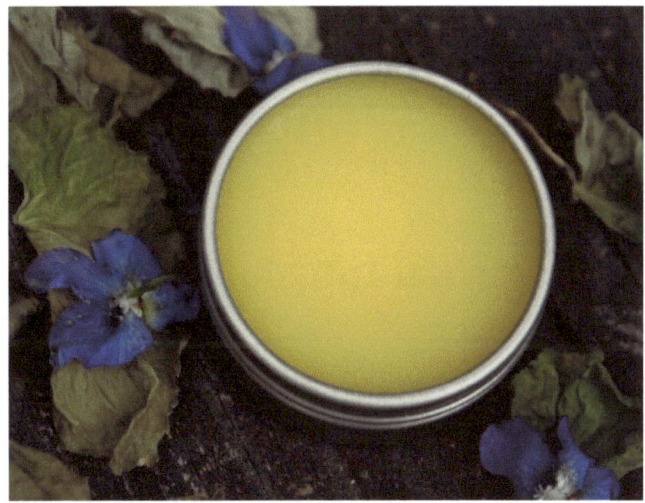

- 3.5 ounces (100 grams) infused violet leaf oil
- 0.5 ounce (15 grams) beeswax

Directions

1. Combine the beeswax and violet leaf oil in a heat-proof jar.
2. Set the jar down into a small saucepan containing an inch or two of water and heat it over a medium-low burner until the beeswax is melted.
3. Remove it from the heat and pour the mixture into tins or small jars. This recipe makes approximately 4 ounces of balm.
4. Massage the balm into your breasts and underarms nightly.

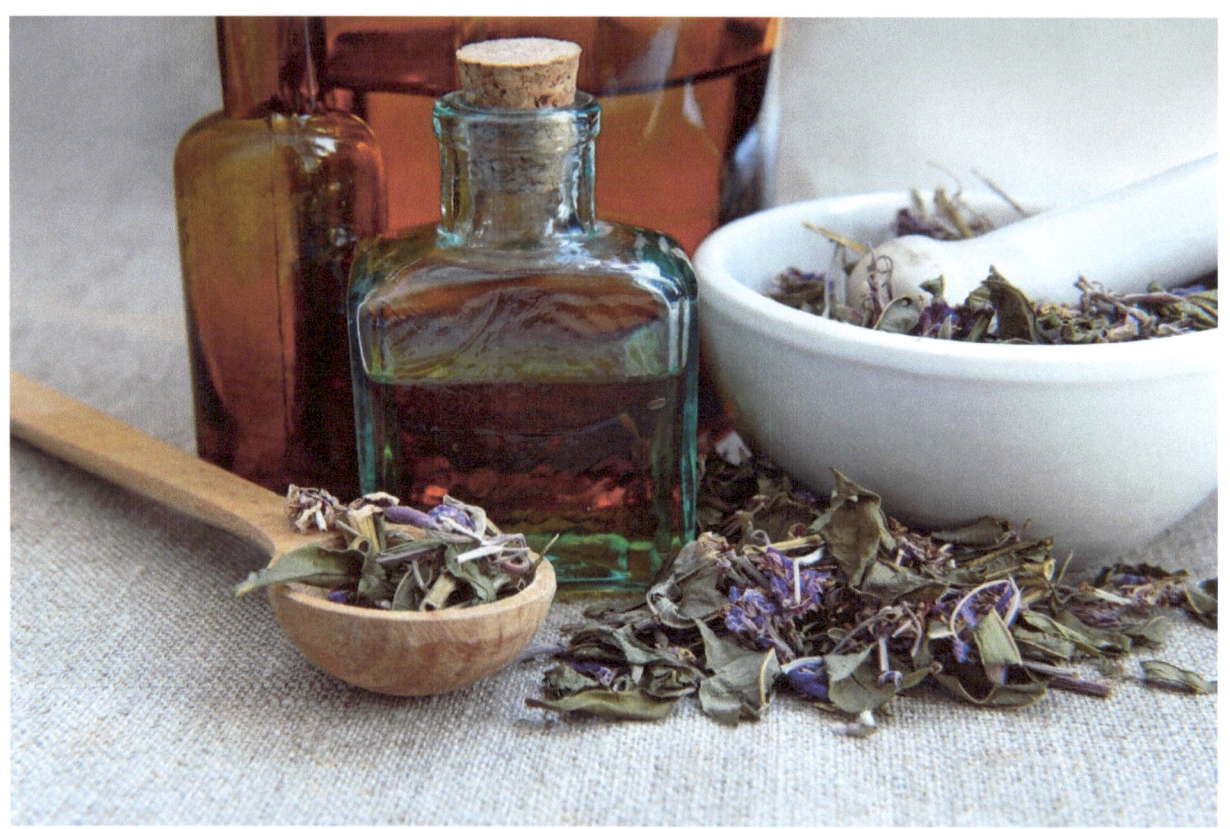

Wise Women's Violet Recipes

Amanda Klenner

Violet Herbal Infusions

I love adding violet leaf to my herbal infusions. Not only does it have a mildly sweet and delightful flavor, but it also adds some extra balancing to common herbs we take as infusions. Here in Colorado, the air is often dry. I see more people suffering from dry constitution and conditions than anything else.

If you know me and my practice, you know I focus a lot on nourishing and supporting the body in its optimal health by helping a person find balance emotionally, physically, and spiritually. Often, nourishing herbal infusions are made with more astringent herbs that can dry the body, like red raspberry leaf, nettle leaf, and dandelion leaf. All of these are drying in nature. I find by combining these nourishing herbs with the soothing demulcent nature of violet leaf, we can help a person become more balanced in constitution.

I also commonly sip on violet leaf infusion all on its own. The flavor is mildly sweet with a little bit of a tannic bite and a nice demulcent soothing quality. When I drink violet leaf infusion, my mouth and throat feel coated and moist without the overbearing sliminess of a marshmallow or slippery elm infusion.

Simple Violet Leaf Infusion

I like this infusion as a soothing, cooling drink for the digestive and respiratory system. I also use it as a topical compress for hot, swollen tissues. It's soothing and encourages healing when used topically on sunburns and contact dermatitis.

Ingredients
- 1 ounce violet leaf (flowers can be used here too)
- 1 quart just-boiled water

Directions
1. Place your violet leaf in a 1-quart glass jar and pour the boiled water over it.
2. Allow this to sit for 4–8 hours. We want to extract the nutritional constituents with the heat, and then let the tea cool to extract the mucilage from the violet leaf.
3. Drink as you like within 48 hours. (This can also be frozen—and labeled—for a quick cooling treat for angry skin, or added as ice cubes to summer drinks for extra soothing and cooling power.)

Nourishing Herbal Infusion with Violet

Nourishing herbal infusions are strong, slow-infused teas meant to be drunk throughout the day for a nutrient-rich boost. You can easily add violet leaf to these nutritious teas. This simple partial substitution helps those of us in dry climates maintain a healthy balance of moisture in the body.

Ingredients

- 1 ounce of a nutritive herb like nettle leaf, red raspberry leaf, red clover, alfalfa leaf, dandelion leaf or root, or burdock root
- $1/4$ ounce violet leaf (plus flower if you like)
- 1 quart just-boiled water

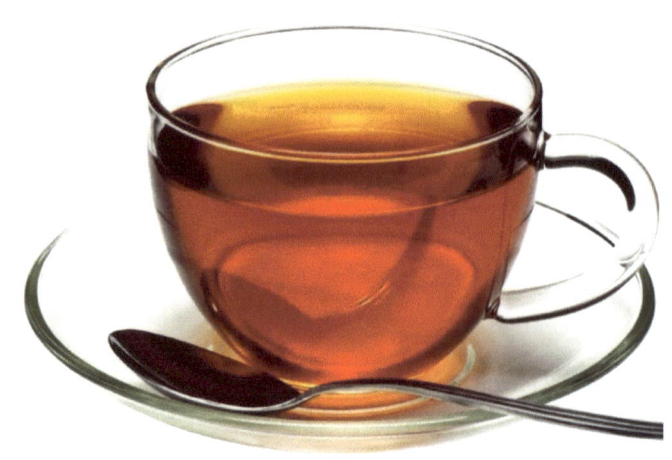

Directions

1. Pour boiled water over the herbs in a glass jar.
2. Steep as described in the previous recipe, for 4–8 hours
3. Drink as you like within 48 hours.

Note: This is not recommended for someone with an overly damp constitution or condition. If your constitution is damp, slimy, and slug-like, violet leaf is not for you!

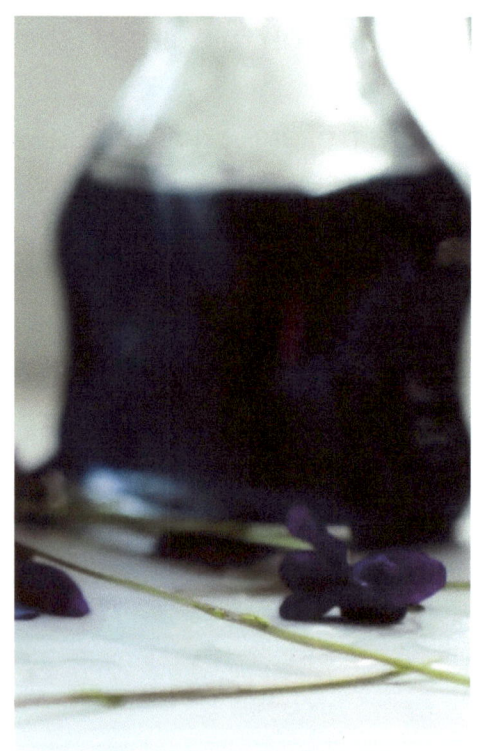

Violet Syrup

Violet leaf (and/or flower) syrup is a common and tasty remedy for coughs and colds, sore throats, and oral burns. I love the combination of the soothing demulcent qualities of violet leaf along with the anti-infective and lymphatic benefits. These qualities make it a soothing and gentle remedy for the whole family!

Cough Syrup (with honey)

This is truly an herb-mamma remedy if there ever was one. Mothers and healers alike have used it commonly across Europe and America for centuries as a simple, soothing, medicine. Other herbs can be added for specific health conditions, but I find a simple violet syrup often does the trick for dry, hot conditions.

Note: Remember, honey is not recommended for use by children under 12 months of age by the FDA. If this is intended for a younger child, replace the honey with raw turbinado sugar or vegetable glycerin.

Ingredients

- 1 C violet leaf (flowers can also be used, and they add a delicious floral note as well as a beautiful purple color)
- 3 C water
- 1 – $1^1/_2$ C honey
- Brandy as a preservative (optional)

Directions

1. Place the violets in a stainless steel or other non-reactive pan and cover them with cool, pure water. Allow this to sit overnight.
2. The next day, simmer the violet leaf in water until the water is reduced to about half the beginning volume ($1^1/_2$ C of decoction)
3. Strain the herbs and squeeze out all the liquid goodness. Compost the herb.
4. In another pot, pan or bowl, add the warm (not boiling and not cold) decoction to the honey and stir well. Do not boil the honey as it will deactivate its enzymes.
5. Add $^1/_2$ C of brandy as a preservative (optional) or refrigerate the syrup. It keeps without alcohol for about 2–3 months in the refrigerator.
6. 1 tsp to 1 Tbsp can be taken as needed to soothe dry, hot conditions of the mouth, throat, lungs, and stomach.

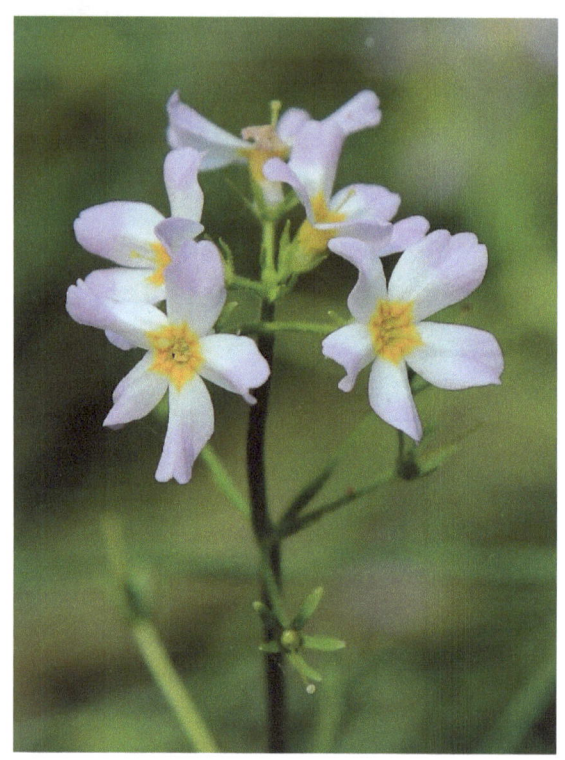

Water Violet Flower Essence

Charis Denny

Not a true violet, water violet (*Hottonia palustris*) does share some similarities with *Viola spp*. Its pretty, delicate, sometimes dual-colored flowers look like violets, for starters. Water violet has a hiding tendency too, like *Viola* violets, but it's the leaves that hide out under water, while the flowers reach up, rising well above the rest of the plant.

Water violet flower essence is indicated for someone who may at first seem like a shrinking violet—shy, withdrawn, easily intimidated. The water violet personality upon better understanding, proves to be more aloof, distant, or even arrogant. He or she will have a demeanor that allows them to deal calmly and capably with whatever life throws at them, but they won't place a lot of emphasis on social relationships or being involved with their community, unless it benefits them directly.

It's not that they are selfish or snobby, it is just that their self-contained nature keeps them from becoming strongly connected with other human beings. People may find them hard to know, and they often lack warm and personable relationships in their lives.

Water violet flower essence can help those for whom it is indicated to recognize the importance of integrating with the people surrounding them—their family, friends, or professional peers, as well as their community at large. It can help them understand how giving of themselves brings to them in return the pleasures of relationship, something that can be difficult for the out-of-balance water violet person to maintain, or to even value.

On the soul level, there is only so far that a person can evolve on their own as an entity separate from everyone else; and water violet flower essence can help emphasize for them the importance of kinship to soul growth.

Water violet flower essence can also help those who take it to attain a more open and involved state of consciousness. When brought into proper balance, a water violet personality can begin not only to connect with the people around them, but also to truly understand the importance of these compassionate connections with others.

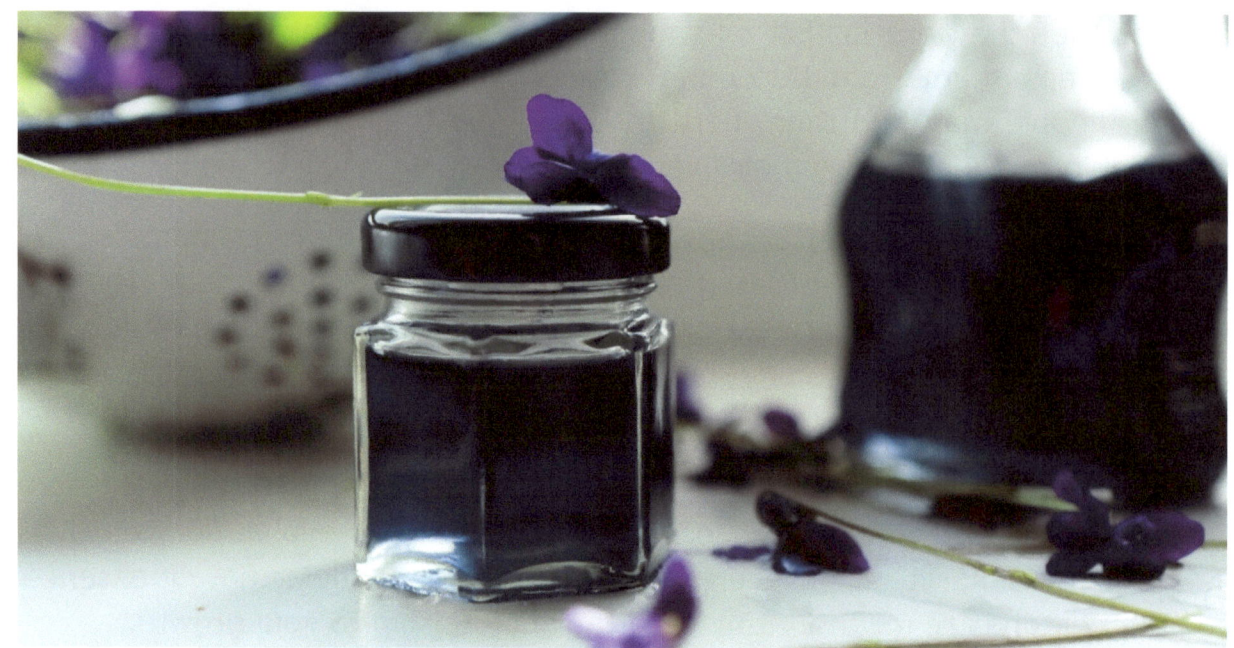

A Taste of Magic: Using Violets in the Kitchen

Erin Smith

There is something about violet's delicate beauty and sweet perfume in early spring that inspires giddiness. Perhaps that's because it's one of the first signs of green lushness after a long winter, but I also think it is part of this little plant's great medicine. Violets have a playful and magical energy about them. They are also delicious!

While I love working with violets medicinally, it's also one of my favorite herbs to work with in the kitchen. Their subtle perfume and sweetness taste as if they are from another world. Any dish with violets will fill the heart and bring smiles.

Violets usually flower from March to May. There are lots of ways to use violet leaf in the kitchen (in a wild-foods pesto, as a salad green, etc.), but the flowers are actually what I use most. Make sure you have *Viola odorata*, which you will know by its fragrance. In fact, you will often smell this species of violet before you see it. Some other violet relatives are edible, but for these recipes, you want the sweet fragrance of the common violet. To capture the most of their fragrance, harvest the fully opened flowers on a sunny day. It is best not to wash the flowers, as it will diminish the flavor and fragrance, so be sure to harvest from an area you know is safe.

Violet flowers are truly a gift from the plant world. Since the flowers are not required for reproduction (violets depend on runners and seed dispersal from later-blooming non-descript flowers for reproduction), you can enjoy as many of the fragrant flowers as you want and not worry about affecting the population. Don't hesitate to enjoy this treat so delightful that some believe it's a gift from the fairies! Here are some of my favorite ways to use violet.

Lemon Scones

This is fit for a fairy queen, and it's a treat I look forward to every spring. The recipe below is the gluten-free version I make, but you can simply substitute regular flour for the flours listed, if you prefer traditional scones.

Scone Ingredients

- 1 C gluten free oat flour
- 1 C gluten free flour mix of choice
- $1/4$ C coconut or date sugar
- 1 tsp baking powder
- 1 tsp baking soda
- $1/4$ tsp sea salt
- 1 stick of grass-fed unsalted butter, cold
- $1/2$ C buttermilk (full fat if you can find it)
- Zest of two lemons

   Note: If you are oat-sensitive, you can substitute another flour, but your scones will be heavier.

Scone Directions

1. Preheat the oven to 350°F (375°F at 3500 feet or higher elevation).
2. In a large bowl or mixer, combine the flour, sugar, baking powder, baking soda, and salt.

3. Add in the stick of butter, cutting off small pieces with a knife. If you're using a mixer, combine the mixture until it resembles fine crumbs. If you are doing this by hand, achieve the same small-crumb effect by cutting through the mixture with two knifes.
4. Add the buttermilk and lemon zest.
5. Blend just until the ingredients are combined.
6. Place the dough onto a floured surface and knead it a few times.
7. Pat it into a ball.
8. Press the dough down until it forms a circle about $1/2$ inch thick.
9. Place the dough circle on a greased baking sheet.
10. With a knife, cut wedges into the circle (as you would a pie) but do not cut all the way through.
11. Bake for 20-25 minutes (12-17 minutes at elevation) or until edges are slightly brown.
12. Serve warm, sliced in half with violet butter (see below).

Violet Butter

Butter Ingredients
- 1 stick of unsalted butter, room temperature
- 1 C fresh violet flowers
- 1 Tbsp (or to taste) maple syrup or honey

Note: I use less than 1 Tbsp of honey because I tend to prefer my butter only slightly sweet so that the taste of the violets stands out. Feel free to experiment, starting small, until it reaches the sweetness you desire.

Butter Directions
1. In a mixer, combine all the ingredients until they're well blended. (It's much easier to use a mixer, but this can be done by hand if needed. It will just take a lot more work to make sure the syrup or honey is evenly blended.)
2. Serve with the scones from the recipe above, or with pancakes, waffles, blueberry muffins, or anything else you think it would go well with!

Note: Leftover violet butter must be stored in the refrigerator and should be used within a few weeks, or the fresh flowers will begin to mold. It can also be frozen and saved for much longer. I always freeze anything I'm not going to eat within a week.

Violet Cordial*

This is a fun and delicious floral cordial that captures the flavor of violets so you can enjoy it for months to come. It is a beautiful magenta color, and it has a nice delicate flavor. A cordial makes a delightful addition to cool summer spritzers, cocktails, ice cream, and so much more.

Adapted from a recipe for Elderflower Cordial by Julie Bruton-Seal and Matthew Seal

Ingredients

- 5 C fresh violet flowers
- $4^1/_2$ C organic raw sugar
- 8 C water
- $3^1/_4$ Tbsp citric acid

Directions

1. Place the sugar and water in a saucepan and bring it to a boil.
2. After it boils for 5 minutes, remove it from the heat and stir, making sure all the sugar has dissolved.
3. Pour the mixture into a large ceramic or glass bowl.
4. Add the citric acid.
5. Add the violet flowers and stir well.
6. Cover with a clean cloth and let sit, unrefrigerated, for 4 days, stirring a bit each day.
7. After 4 days, strain through a cheesecloth and bottle.

Your cordial will last in the refrigerator for months. To store it longer, you can also freeze it. To enjoy it, add a little bit (exact amount can be to taste) to sparkling water. Other ideas include adding a bit to fruit salads, cocktails, fruit compotes, etc.

Note: I've tried to make this recipe with honey instead of sugar and it doesn't work as well. The strong flavor of honey overpowers the delicate flavor of the violets. While it seems like a lot of sugar, keep in mind that you are only using a small amount of the finished cordial each time. The sugar also acts as a preservative.

Violet-Infused Honey

This is super easy to make, and it offers another delicious way to capture violets for year-round enjoyment.

Ingredients
- Fresh violet flowers
- Raw honey

Directions
1. Fill a glass jar with fresh violet flowers.
2. Pour raw honey over the flowers until they're covered.
3. Use a chopstick or spoon to stir and push the flowers down so they all sit below the surface of the honey.
4. Allow to stand for 3-4 weeks. It's normal for the flowers to rise to the top. Simply turn the jar over to mix it up, or open it occasionally and stir with a spoon.
5. Enjoy! (There's no need to strain it; use it with the flowers in it.)

Violet Syrup (with sugar)

Syrup is similar to a cordial, but the flavor is different. It's sweeter and less delicate. The color is different too—purplish-blue, instead of magenta, and, syrups tend to be thicker than cordials. Syrups are commonly used medicinally (see Amanda's cough syrup recipe, page 31), but there are all sorts of creative ways to use them in the kitchen too: Try it in summer drinks and desserts, as well as pancakes and waffles, yogurt, and fruit salad.

Ingredients

- 3 C filtered or spring water
- 2 C fresh violet flowers
- About 2 C raw sugar

Directions

1. Bring the water to a boil and then remove it from the heat.
2. Add the fresh violet flowers and stir.
3. Cover the pan and allow it to stand until cool (the longer the better). The infusion will be a beautiful purplish blue color.
4. When it's cooled, strain the infusion into a large measuring cup or bowl, setting the violet flowers aside.
5. Gently reheat the infusion in a saucepan on medium heat.
6. Note how much liquid you have and add an equal amount of raw sugar (if you have 2 C violet infusion, add 2 C sugar).
7. Stir the sugar in until it dissolves.
8. Remove from heat.
9. The sugar acts as a preservative, but if you want the syrup to last longer, add $1/4$ part brandy or vodka. This is optional.
10. Bottle and store it in the refrigerator.

Note: If you have a favorite recipe for making syrups, that will work fine too. However, because of violet's delicate nature, I find that an infusion is better than a decoction, so don't boil the flowers.

Berries with Violet Cream

Berries and cream in any form is my favorite dessert. You can make what seems like a simple dish just a bit snazzier by infusing violets in the cream.

Ingredients

- 1 pint whipping cream or thick cream of your choice
- $1/4$ to $1/2$ C fresh violet flowers

Directions

1. Pour the cream into a bowl.

2. Add the fresh violet flowers.

3. Stir to make sure the flowers are covered in the cream.

4. Allow them to infuse in the refrigerator overnight.

5. When you're ready to use the cream, strain out the flowers, add a bit of honey or maple syrup (to taste), and whip as usual. This works great with roses too!

Violet Ice Cubes

Another simple and fun way to use violets is to make ice cubes that perfectly frame and preserve each little delicate flower.

Ingredients

- Clean, filtered water
- Violet flowers

Directions

1. Fill an ice cube tray with filtered water.

2. Place one fresh flower in each cube and push it down with a knife or a chopstick.

3. Freeze the cubes and add them to your favorite spring and summer beverages.

This works well with any edible flower.

Decorate with Violets

Sometimes simple is best. During violet season, I also add fresh violet flowers to lots of dishes. They look and taste great sprinkled on salads, oatmeal, desserts, and fruit salads!

References and Resources

Monograph

Cited

[1] Susun S. Weed, *Breast Cancer? Breast Health!* (Ash Tree Publishing, 1996), 46.

[2] Susun S. Weed, *Healing Wise* (Ash Tree Publishing, 1989), 243

[3] Anne McIntyre, *Flower Power* (Henry Holt & Company, Inc., 1996), 238

[4] Weed, *Healing*, 246

[5] McIntyre, *Flower*, 240

[6] Richard Mabey, Michael McIntyre, Pamela Michael, Gail Duff, John Stevens, Jane Reynolds, Nigel Hawtin, *The New Age Herbalist: How to Use Herbs for Healing, nutrition, Body Care, and Relaxation* (Fireside, 1988), 125

[7] Earnest Leaverton, *In the Garden of the Heart* (J. F. Tapley Company, 1919), 179

[8] Weed, *Healing*, 244

[9] McIntyre, *Flower*, 238

[10] Kiva Rose, "Shy Violets: For Grace, Fluidity and Sweetness," *The Medicine Woman's Roots*, 2007. http://bearmedicineherbals.com/shy-violets-for-grace-fluidity   and-sweetness.html

[11] Jim McDonald, "Violet Herb," *Methow Valley Herbs*, 2014. http://www.methowvalleyherbs.com/2014/03/violet-herb-guest-post-by-jim-mcdonald.html

[12] David Hoffman, *The Complete Illustrated Herbal* (Element Books, 1996), 162

[13] McIntyre, *Flower*, 238

[14] Mrs. M. Grieves, *A Modern Herbal* (Random House, 1973), 839

[15] Weed, *Breast*, 115

[16] Weed, *Breast*, 289

[17] Hoffman, *Ill. Herbal*, 163

[18] Weed, *Healing*, 240

[19] Ed Smith, *Therapeutic Herb Manual*, 1999 p. 53

Uncited

Francois Couplan, Ph.D., The Encyclopedia of Edible Plants of North American, Keats Publishing, 1998

Sharol Tilgner, N.D., Herbal Medicine from the Heart of the Earth, Wise Acres Press, Inc., 1999

Rosalee de la Forêt, "Emerging From Winter To Find Violet," Methow Valley Herbs, 2010.
http://www.methowvalleyherbs.com/2010/02/emerging-from-winter-to-find-violet.html

A Glossary of Herbalism

Nina Katz

Do you feel befuddled by all of those terms? Are you curious about what a menstruum might be, or a nervine? Wondering what the exact difference is between an infusion and a decoction? Or what it means to macerate? Read on; the herbalist lexicographer will reveal it all!

Ad*ap*togen	n.	An herb that enhances one's ability to thrive despite stress. Eleuthero, or Siberian Ginseng *(Eleutherococcus senticosus)* is a well-known adaptogen.
*Ae*rial *parts*	n. pl.	The parts of a plant that grow above ground. Stems, leaves, and flowers are all aerial parts, in contrast to roots and rhizomes.
*Al*terative	n.	An herb that restores the body to health gradually and sustainably by strengthening one or more of the body's systems, such as the digestive or lymphatic system, or one or more of the vital organs, such as the liver or kidneys. Burdock *(Arctium lappa)* is an alternative.
	adj.	Restoring health gradually, as by strengthening one or more of the body's systems or vital organs.
Anthel*mintic*	n.	A substance that eliminates intestinal worms.
Anthel*min*	adj.	Being of or concerning a substance that eliminates intestinal worms.
A*nti*-ca*tarr*hal	n.	A substance that reduces or slows down the production of phlegm.
	adj.	Being of or concerning a substance that reduces or slows down the production of phlegm.
Anti-emetic	n.	A substance that treats nausea. Ginger *(Zingiber officinale)* is anti-emetic.
	adj.	Being of or concerning a substance that treats nausea.

Anti-microbial	n.	An herb or a preparation that helps the body fight off microbial infections, whether viral, bacterial, fungal, or parasitic. Herbal anti-microbials may do this by killing the microbes directly, but more often achieve this by enhancing immune function and helping the body to fight off disease and restore balance.
	adj.	Being of or concerning an herb or a preparation that helps the body fight off microbial infections.
Aperient	n.	A gentle laxative, such as seaweed, plantain seeds *(Plantago spp.)*, or ripe bananas.
	adj.	Being of or concerning a gentle laxative.
Aphrodisiac	n.	A substance that enhances sexual interest or desire.
	adj.	Being of or relating to a substance that enhances sexual interest or desire.
Astringent	n.	A food, herb, or preparation that causes tissues to constrict, or draw in. Astringents help stop bleeding, diarrhea, and other conditions in which some bodily substance is flowing excessively. Some astringents, such as Wild Plantain *(Plantago major)*, draw so powerfully that they can remove splinters.
	adj	Causing tissues to constrict, and thereby helping to stop excessive loss of body fluids.
Bitter	n.	A food, herb, or preparation that stimulates the liver and digestive organs through its bitter flavor. Dandelion *(Taraxacum officinale)* and Gentian *(Gentiana lutea)* are both bitters. Also called *digestive bitter.*
Carminative	n.	A food, herb, or preparation that reduces the buildup or facilitates the release of intestinal gases. Cardamom *(Amomum spp. and Elettaria spp)* and Fennel *(Foeniculum vulgare)* are carminatives.
	adj.	Characterized as reducing the buildup or

facilitating the release of intestinal gases.

*Ca*rrier Oil	n.	A non-medicinal oil, such as olive or sesame oil, used to dilute an essential oil.
Ca*tarrh*	n.	An inflammation of the mucous membranes resulting in an overproduction of phlegm.
Com*pound*	v.	To create a medicinal formula using two or more components.
	n.	An herbal preparation consisting of two or more herbs.
*Com*press	n.	A topical preparation consisting of a cloth soaked in a liquid herbal extract, such as an infusion or decoction, and applied, usually warm or hot, to the body. A washcloth soaked in a hot ginger decoction and applied to a sore muscle is a compress.
De*coct*	v.	To prepare by simmering in water, usually for at least 20 minutes. One usually decocts barks, roots, *rhizomes*, hard seeds, twigs, and nuts.
De*coct*ion	n.	An herbal preparation made by simmering the plant parts in water, usually for at least 20 minutes.
De*mul*cent	n.	An herb with a smooth, slippery texture soothing to the mucous membranes, i.e. the tissues lining the respiratory and digestive tracts. Slippery elm *(Ulmus rubra)*, marshmallow root *(Althaea officinalis)*, and sassafras *(Sassafras albidum, Sassafras officinale)* are all demulcents.
	adj.	Having a smooth, slippery texture that soothes the mucous membranes.
Diapho*retic*	n.	An herb or preparation that opens the pores of the skin, facilitates sweat, and thereby lowers fevers. In Chinese medicine, diaphoretics are said to "release the exterior."□ Yarrow *(Achillea millefolium)* is a diaphoretic.
	adj.	Opening the pores, facilitating sweat, and thereby lowering fevers.
Di*gestive*	n.	An herb, food, or preparation that promotes the

		healthy breakdown, assimilation, and elimination of food, as by gently stimulating the digestive tract in preparation for a meal. Dandelion *(Taraxacum officinale)* and bitter salad greens are digestives.
	adj. 1	Concerning or being part of the bodily system responsible for the breakdown, assimilation, and elimination of food.
	adj. 2	Promoting the healthy breakdown, assimilation, and/or elimination of food.
Diuretic	n.	A substance that facilitates or increases urination. Diuretics can improve kidney function and treat swelling. Excessive use of diuretics can also tax the kidneys. Stinging Nettles *(Urtica dioica)*, cucumbers, and coffee are all diuretics.
	adj.	Facilitating or increasing urination.
Emmenagogue	n.	An herb or preparation that facilitates or increases menstrual flow. Black cohosh *(Cimicifuga racemosa)* is an emmenagogue. Emmenagogues are generally contraindicated in pregnancy.
	adj.	Facilitating or increasing menstrual flow.
Essential *Oil*	n.	An oil characterized by a strong aroma, strong taste, the presence of terpines, and by vaporizing in low temperatures. Essential oils are components of many plants, and when isolated, make fairly strong medicine used primarily externally or for inhalation, and usually not safe for internal use.
	n. 1	A preparation made by chemically removing the soluble parts of a substance into a solvent or menstruum. Herbalists often make extracts using water, alcohol, glycerin, vinegar, oil, or combinations of these. Infusions, medicinal vinegars, tinctures, decoctions, and medicinal oils are all extracts.
	n. 2	A tincture.
Extract	v.	To remove the soluble parts of a substance into a solvent or menstruum by chemical means.
Febrifuge	n.	An herb or preparation that lowers fevers. Yarrow *(Achillea millefolium)*, ginger *(Zingiber officinale)*, and boneset *(Eupatorium perfoliatum)* are all febrifuges.
Galactagogue	n.	A substance that increases the production or flow

		of milk; a remedy that aids lactation. Nettle *(Urtica dioica)* and hops *(Humulus lupulus)* are galactagogues.
*Glan*dular	n.	A substance that treats the adrenal, thyroid, or other glands. Nettle seeds *(Urtica dioica)* are a glandular for the adrenals.
	adj.	Relating to or treating the adrenal, thyroid, or other glands.
He*pa*tic	n.	A substance that treats the liver. Dandelion *(Taraxacum officinale)* is a hepatic.
Hyp*n*otic	n.	An herb or preparation that induces sleep. Chamomile *(Matricaria recutita)* and valerian *(Valeriana officinale)* are both hypnotics.
	adj.	Inducing sleep.
In*fuse*	v.	To prepare by steeping in water, especially hot water, straining, and squeezing the marc.
In*fus*ion	n.	A preparation made by first steeping one or more plants or plant parts in water, most often hot water, and then straining the plant material, usually while squeezing the marc. An infusion extracts the flavor, aroma, and water-soluble nutritional and medicinal constituents into the water.
Long In*fus*ion	n.	An infusion that steeps for three or more hours. Long infusions often steep overnight.
Lym*ph*atic	n.	A substance that stimulates the circulation of lymph or *tonifies* the vessels or organs involved in the circulation or storage of lymph.
*Ma*cerate	v.	To soak a plant or plant parts in a *menstruum* so as to extract the medicinal constituents chemically.
Marc	n.	The plant material left after straining a preparation made by steeping, simmering, or macerating.
*Men*struum	n.	*(Plural, **menstrua** or **menstruums**.)* The solvent used to extract the medicinal and/or nutritional constituents from a plant. Water, alcohol, vinegar, and glycerin are among the more common menstrua.
*Mu*cilage	n.	A thick, slippery, *demulcent* substance produced

by a plant or microorganism.

*Muci*laginous	n.	Having or producing mucilage; *demulcent.* Okra, marshmallow root *(Althaea officinalis)*, sassafras *(Sassafras albidum, Sassafras officinale)*, and slippery elm *(Ulmus rubra)* are all mucilaginous.
*Ner*vine	n.	An herb or preparation that helps with problems traditionally associated with the nerves, such as mental health issues, insomnia, and pain.
	adj.	Helping with problems traditionally associated with the nerves, such as mental health issues, insomnia, and pain.
Pectoral	n.	A substance that treats the lungs or the respiratory system.
*Poul*tice	n.	A mass of plant material or other substances, usually mashed, gnashed, moistened, or heated, and placed directly on the skin. Sometimes covered by a cloth or adhesive. A plantain *(Plantago spp.)* poultice can draw splinters out.
*Rhiz*ome	n.	A usually horizontal stem that grows underground, is marked by nodes from which roots grow down, and branches out to produce a network of new plants growing up from the nodes.
Salve	[sæv] n.	A soothing ointment prepared from beeswax combined with oil, usually medicinal oil, and used in topical applications.
Short Infusion	n.	An *infusion* that steeps for a relatively short period of time, usually 5-30 minutes.
Sedative	n.	A substance that calms and facilitates sleep. Valerian *(Valeriana officinale)* is a sedative.
Sedative	adj.	Calming and facilitating sleep.
*Sim*ple	n.	An herbal preparation, such as a tincture or decoction, made from one herb alone.
*Simp*ler	n.	An herbalist who prepares and recommends primarily *simples* rather than compounds.
Spp.	abbr. n.pl.	Species. *Used to indicate more than one species in the same botanical family. Echinacea spp. includes*

both *Echinacea purpurea* and *Echinacea angustifolium*, among other species. *Plantago spp.* includes both *Plantago major* and *Plantago lanceolata.*

Stimulant	n.	An herb or preparation that increases the activity level in an organ or body system. Echinacea *(Echinacea spp.)* is an immunostimulant; it stimulates the immune system. Cayenne *(Capsicum spp.)* is a circulatory stimulant. Rosemary is a stimulant to the nervous, digestive, and circulatory systems.
Sudorific	adj.	Increasing sweat or facilitating the release of sweat; cf. *diaphoretic.*
Syrup	n.	A sweet liquid preparation, often made by adding honey or sugar to a decoction.
Tea	n.	A drink made by steeping a plant or plant parts, especially *Camellia sinensis.*
Tisane	n.	An herbal beverage made by decoction or short infusion and not prepared from the tea plant *(Camellia sinensis).*
Tincture	n.	A preparation made by macerating one or more plants or plant parts in a *menstruum,* usually alcohol or glycerin, straining, and squeezing the *marc* in order to extract the chemical constituents into the *menstruum.*
	v.	To prepare by *macerating* in a *menstruum,* straining, and squeezing the marc in order to extract the chemical constituents.
Tonic	n.	A substance that strengthens one or more organs or systems, or the entire organism. Stinging nettle *(Urtica dioica)* is a general tonic, as well as a specific kidney, liver, and hair tonic. Red raspberry leaf *(Rubus idaeus)* is a reproductive tonic; Mullein *(Verbascum thapsus)* is a respiratory tonic.
Tonify	v.	To strengthen. Nettle *(Urtica dioica)* tonifies the entire body.
Volatile Oil	n.	An oil characterized by volatility, or rapid vaporization at relatively low temperatures; cf. *essential oil.*
Vulnerary	n.	A substance that soothes and heals wounds. Comfrey *(Symphytum officinale)* is an excellent vulnerary.

adj.   Being or concerning a substance that soothes and heals wounds.

Disclaimer

Nothing provided by Natural Living Mamma LLC, Natural Herbal Living Magazine, or Herb Box should be considered medical advice. Nothing included here is approved by the FDA and the information provided herein is for informational purposes only. Always consult a botanically knowledgeable medical practitioner before starting any course of treatment, especially if you are pregnant, breastfeeding, on any medications, or have any health problems. Natural Living Mamma LLC is not liable for any action or inaction you take based on the information provided here.